The Art of
EDIBLE
FLOWERS

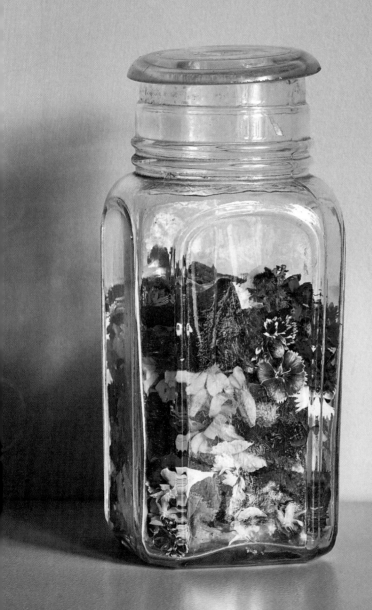

The Art of
EDIBLE
FLOWERS

Recipes and ideas for floral salads,
drinks, desserts and more

Rebecca Sullivan

photography by Nassima Rothacker

Kyle Books

For my grandad, graham.
May he be surrounded by flowers in heaven.

First published in Great Britain in 2018
by Kyle Cathie Limited
Part of Octopus Publishing Group Limited
Carmelite House, 50 Victoria Embankment
London EC4Y 0DZ
www.kylebooks.co.uk

10 9 8 7 6 5 4 3 2 1

ISBN 978 0 85783 476 8

Project Editor: Tara O'Sullivan
Copy Editor: Anne Sheasby
Editorial Assistant: Sarah Kyle
Designer: Laura Woussen
Photographer: Nassima Rothacker
Illustrator: Chrissy Lau
Stylists: Rebecca Sullivan and Rachel de Thample
Prop Stylist: Agathe Gits
Production: Lisa Pinnell

A Cataloguing in Publication record for this title is
available from the British Library.

Colour reproduction by ALTA London
Printed and bound in China by 1010 International
Printing Ltd

The information and advice contained in this book are
intended as a general guide to using plants and are not
specific to individuals or their particular circumstances.
Many plant substances, whether sold as foods or
as medicines and used externally or internally, can
cause an allergic reaction in some people. Neither
the author nor the publishers can be held responsible
for claims arising from the inappropriate use of any
remedy or healing regime. Do not attempt self-diagnosis
or self-treatment for serious or long-term conditions
before consulting a medical professional or qualified
practitioner. Do not undertake any self-treatment while
taking other prescribed drugs or receiving therapy
without first seeking professional guidance. Always seek
medical advice if any symptoms persist.

CONTENTS

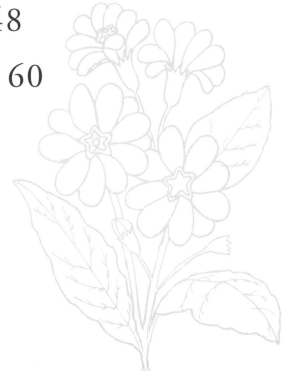

Introduction

Flowers remind me of my grandad. He was so very proud of his garden, and the smell of a rose conjures up many happy memories of my childhood. Not just roses either. In the peak of summer, whenever I see a honeysuckle creeping along someone's fence, I have to stop, pick a flower and eat its little sweet treat inside. For as long as I can remember, I have been rather obsessed with eating the pretty petals of any plant I can. Well, at least until I learned by trial and error of the nasty kind, that not all pretty things can be eaten.

Flowers can make a dull dish beautiful in an instant with an array of colour, they can add flavour and texture, but some of them also pack a powerful medicinal punch too.

It's rather in vogue to eat flowers at the moment and it has been a trend that has gone in and out of fashion for many a decade. But it is actually something that has been around for longer than you would think – centuries, in fact. Eating flowers is not really something that can sustain you, nutritionally speaking, but it makes a wonderful addition to savoury and sweet dishes and can take a rather dull salad to somewhat Michelin-star heights by way of plating it up prettily. If you think about it, flowers in food are all around us. We use hops for beer, roses to make rose water, chrysanthemums to make rice cakes, calendula is used for medicine, and lavender covers the south of France to be used in many traditional dishes. Sure, growing perfectly perfumed roses and fields of lavender isn't feasible for those of us without the land or green thumbs to do so, but a few planter boxes of nasturtiums, calendula and geranium on the balcony are doable. Trust me, I have friends who have been known to kill a terrarium that can keep those few things alive. And if growing isn't your thing, then make friends with your neighbours and swap a bunch of roses for a jar of pickled peonies.

But before we all start plating up every flower in sight, it is important to do some research and follow a few rules, so on the following pages you'll find a little straight-forward guide to edible flowers. Once you know your stuff, don't forget to eat pretty and plate up an edible rainbow.

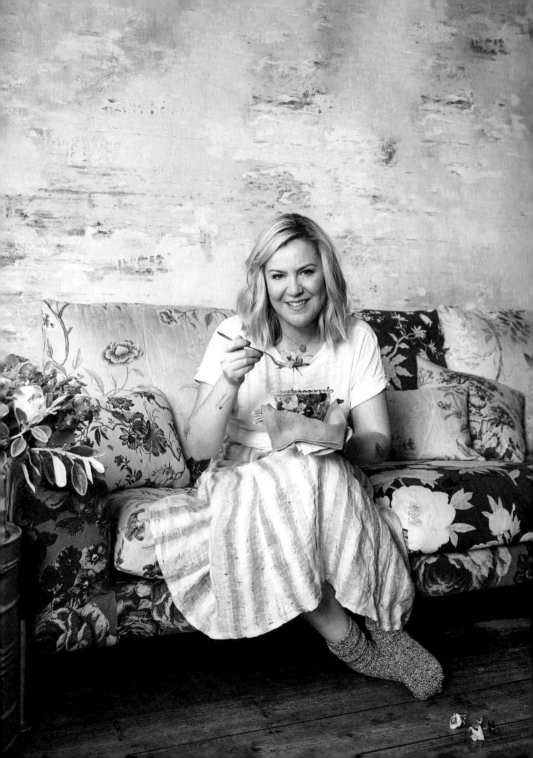

Picking & storing

The most important thing to consider is safety. Do your research. I have compiled a list of some of the most commonly available edible flowers, but there are many more than this. Identify the flower more than once before you eat it and always double and triple check that they have not been sprayed or are so close to a road that they may have been over-polluted by passing traffic.

- When identifying a plant, use a photo or illustration, and make sure you know how to use it and which part is edible (some plants are not entirely edible), as well as the scientific name for the flower. Eat flowers only when you are positive they are edible.

- Remember when picking flowers to be respectful. Leave some for biodiversity and for the plant's longevity. If foraging, this is extremely important.

- Harvest in the morning and after any early dew has dried out, as flowers contain more water at this time. Pick when the flower opens.

- Pick the flowers and place on top of kitchen paper in an airtight container, laying the flowers flat in a single layer. Use multiple containers as opposed to piling them all in one. Store in the fridge.

- Use a delicate pastry brush to brush off any residue or insects from the flowers and do this outdoors so the bugs can go on their merry way.

- If you have pollen allergies, always remove the stamens or pistils from flowers before eating.

- Wash all flowers thoroughly before you eat them.

- Introduce flowers into your diet in small quantities, one species at a time. This is especially important if you have allergies.

- Eat only the flower petals for safety's sake as other parts are often inedible.

- Do not eat flowers from florists, nurseries or garden centres. In many cases, these flowers have been treated with pesticides not intended for food crops.

- Do not eat flowers picked from the side of the road. Once again, possible herbicide use eliminates these flowers from being suitable for edible use.

Edible flowers list

Below are just some of the edible flowers you can experiment with in your dishes.

alliums

alpine pink

angelica – *Angelica archangelica*

arugula (rocket flower)

banana blossoms

bergamot or bee balm – *Monarda*

borage – *Borago officinalis*

burnet

calendula – *Calendula officinalis*

carnation

chamomile – *Matricaria chamomilla*, *Chamaemelum nobile*

chervil – *Anthriscus cerefolium*

chicory – *Cichorium intybus*

chrysanthemum

citrus flower

clover – *Trifolium pratense* (specifically red clover)

common elder – *Sambucus nigra*

cornflower – *Centaurea cyanus*

cowslip – *Primula veris*

culinary herb flowers, such as basil *(Ocimum basilicum)*, borage, chamomile and chive

daisy – *Bellis perennis*

dandelion – *Taraxacum officinale*

day lily (acts as a diuretic, so in moderation)

dianthus (petals only)

fennel flower – *Foeniculum vulgare*

fuchsia

gardenia

geranium (not citronelle variety)

ginger flower

gladiolus

hibiscus

hollyhock

honeysuckle (warning: its berries are highly poisonous) – *Lonicera periclymenum, L.*

caprifolium OR *Lonicera*

hops – *Humulus lupulus*

hyssop – *Hyssopus officinalis impatiens*

jasmine (not false jasmine) – *Jasminum officinale*

lavender

lemon verbena flower

lilac – *Syringa spp.*

marjoram

mock orange

mustard flowers

nasturtium – *Trapaeolum majus*

okra flower

orchid

pansy and viola

pea (not ornamental sweet peas, they are poisonous)

peony

pineapple guava

primrose – *Primula vulgaris*

Queen Anne's lace (don't confuse with wild hemlock, which is highly poisonous)

radish flower

rose – *Rosa* spp.

rose geranium – *Perlargonium graveolens*

saffron

sage – *Salvia officinalis*

snap dragon

squash blossom

sunflower

sweet violet

tiger lily

tulip petals (some people are allergic, so if you get a rash when touching them, don't eat them)

violet – *Viola odorata*

wood sorrel, pink and yellow (sower sob)

yucca

See overleaf for a visual guide to some of the flowers I use most in my cooking.

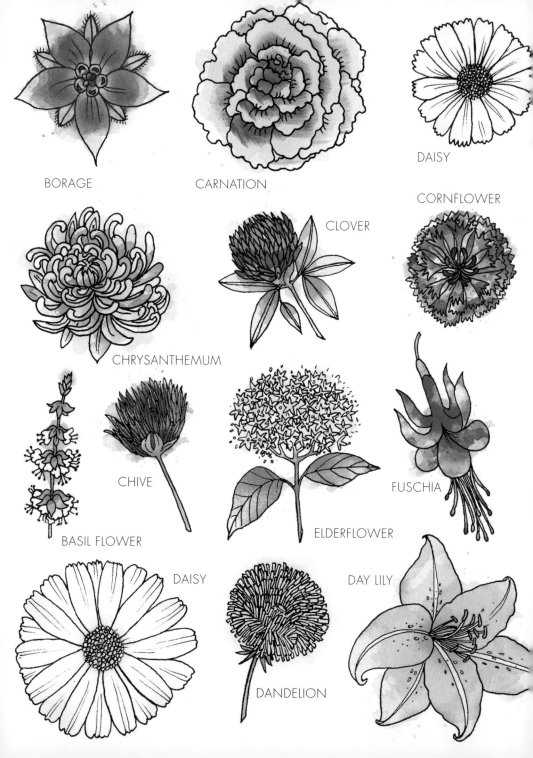

BORAGE

CARNATION

DAISY

CORNFLOWER

CLOVER

CHRYSANTHEMUM

CHIVE

ELDERFLOWER

FUSCHIA

BASIL FLOWER

DAISY

DANDELION

DAY LILY

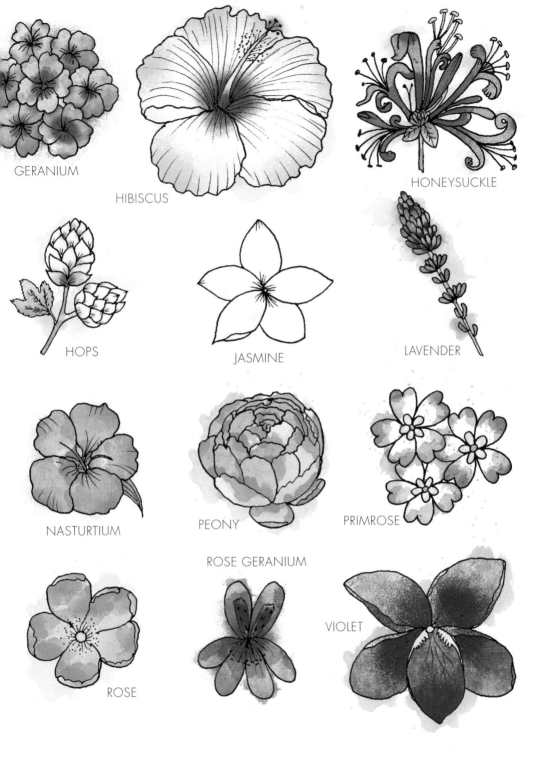

GERANIUM

HIBISCUS

HONEYSUCKLE

HOPS

JASMINE

LAVENDER

NASTURTIUM

PEONY

PRIMROSE

ROSE GERANIUM

ROSE

VIOLET

Chapter One
drinks

Floral syrups six ways

Floral syrups are useful and delicious. They are great to have on hand for when unexpected guests pop in and you have nothing but wine to offer (tragedy in itself!). Perfect for feeling like you're having a grown-up drink when you're trying not to have a grown-up drink.

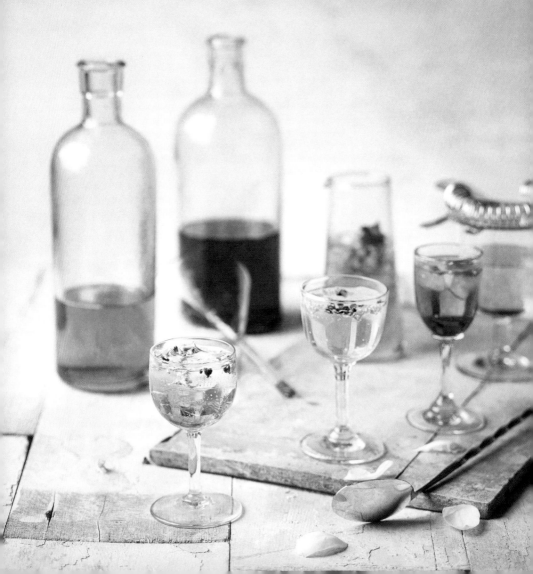

Rose Syrup

MAKES 750ML

250g fresh rose petals, unsprayed – try to choose ones that really smell of roses

500g caster sugar

750ml water

juice of 1 lemon

1–2 teaspoons (depending on how strong you want it) culinary lavender (dried lavender)

sterilised 1 litre jar or bottle

Place the rose petals in a bowl with the sugar and stir to mix, then cover with a tea towel. Leave overnight.

The next day, transfer the rose petal/sugar mixture to a medium saucepan, add the water and stir until the sugar dissolves. Bring to the boil over a high heat, then reduce the heat and simmer for a few minutes. Stir in the lemon juice and lavender.

Strain into a hot sterilised jar, seal and cool. Label and store in a cool, dark place for up to 6 months. Once opened, store in the fridge. Use in cocktails or serve with soda water.

Lavender Syrup

MAKES 750ML

1 teaspoon culinary lavender

500g caster sugar

750ml water

juice of 1 lemon

sterilised 1 litre jar or bottle

Place the lavender in a bowl with the sugar and stir to mix, then cover with a tea towel. Leave overnight.

The next day, transfer the lavender/sugar mixture to a medium saucepan, add the water and stir until the sugar dissolves. Bring to the boil over a high heat, then reduce the heat and simmer for a few minutes. Stir in the lemon juice.

Strain into a hot sterilised jar, seal and cool. Label and store in a cool, dark place for up to 6 months. Once opened, store in the fridge. Use in cocktails or serve with soda water.

Elderflower Syrup

MAKES 1 LITRE

30 fresh elderflower heads
1 litre boiling water
750g caster sugar
juice of 3 lemons

sterilised 1 litre jar or bottle

Place the elderflower heads in a large heatproof bowl, then pour over the boiling water. Cover with a tea towel and leave overnight at room temperature.

The next day, strain into a saucepan. Stir in the sugar and lemon juice, then heat gently, stirring until the sugar has dissolved. Bring to a simmer and continue to simmer for a few minutes.

Pour into a hot sterilised jar, seal and cool. Label and store in a cool, dark place for up to 6 months. Once opened, store in the fridge. Use in cocktails or serve with soda water.

Violet Syrup

MAKES 400ML

4 handfuls fresh violets
375ml boiling water
500g caster sugar
1 teaspoon lemon juice (optional)

sterilised 500ml jar or bottle

Place the violets in a heatproof bowl, then pour over the boiling water. Cover with a tea towel and leave overnight at room temperature.

The next day, strain into a saucepan, squishing the violets as you go. Stir in the sugar and heat slowly until very gently simmering, stirring. Don't boil, just heat until the sugar dissolves. Turn off the heat and add the lemon juice if you want purple liquid. Leave out the juice and it will stay blue.

Pour into a hot sterilised jar, seal and cool. Label and store in a cool, dark place for up to 6 months. Once opened, store in the fridge. Use in cocktails or serve with soda water.

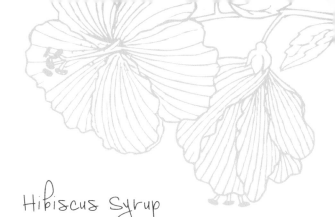

Hibiscus Syrup

MAKES 500ML

480ml water
340g caster sugar
1 handful dried whole hibiscus
  flowers
juice of ½ lemon

sterilised 500ml jar or bottle

Place the water and sugar in a saucepan and bring to the boil, stirring initially to dissolve the sugar. Turn off the heat and add the hibiscus flowers. Set aside for 30 minutes. Stir in the lemon juice.

Strain into a sterilised jar, seal and cool. Label and store in a cool, dark place for up to 6 months. Once opened, store in the fridge. Use in cocktails or serve with soda water.

Fennel flower Syrup

MAKES 1 LITRE

20 fennel flower heads
1 litre boiling water
750g caster sugar
juice of 3 lemons

sterilised 1 litre jar or bottle

Place the fennel flowers in a large heatproof bowl, then pour over the boiling water. Cover with a tea towel and leave overnight at room temperature.

The next day, strain into a saucepan. Stir in the sugar and lemon juice, then heat gently, stirring until the sugar has dissolved. Bring to a simmer and continue to simmer for a few minutes.

Pour into a hot sterilised jar, seal and cool. Label and store in a cool, dark place for up to 6 months. Once opened, store in the fridge. Use in cocktails or serve with soda water.

Floral bitters

A most wonderful addition to any cocktail that needs bitters, but also a wonderful tonic for health. The herbs and flowers in these bitters have many medicinal benefits, and if you can sneak in a tablespoonful per day (if possible) when you're run down, it acts as a wonderful pick-me-up.

MAKES 500ML

- 1 pink grapefruit
- 1 orange
- 40g dried juniper berries
- 20g dried whole hibiscus flowers
- 4 tablespoons dried rose petals
- 1½ teaspoons dried culinary lavender
- 1 tablespoon dried elderflower or elderberry
- 8 star anise
- 2 tablespoons dried mint
- 2 teaspoons ground white pepper
- 2 tablespoons honey
- 250ml brandy

sterilised 500ml jar or bottle

Cut the grapefruit and orange into squares and add to a sterilised jar, along with all the other ingredients. Seal and shake well. Label and store in a cool, dark place for up to six weeks to infuse. Strain into a clean jar. Label and store in a cool, dark place for up to 2 years. Use 1–2 tablespoons in your drinks as a bitter flavouring.

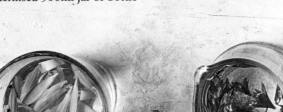
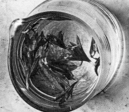
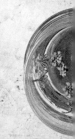

Floral waters

Not only do these smell delightful, they are a great addition to many desserts and baking recipes. If you don't get through them for baking, they make a lovely little face spritz too. Feel free to play around with the flower combinations and add more flowers if you have an abundance.

MAKES 250ML

200ml filtered water
6 tablespoons fresh or dried edible
flowers of your choice (such
as geranium, rose, lavender,
lily or jasmine)

sterilised 250ml jar or bottle

Bring the water to the boil in a small saucepan. Place the flowers in a heatproof bowl. Pour over the boiling water and cover with a plate to weight it down. Leave to infuse overnight at room temperature.

Strain the water into a sterilised jar, then seal and store in the fridge for up to 6 months. Use as needed.

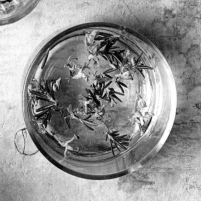

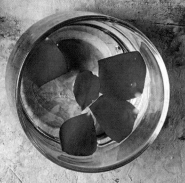

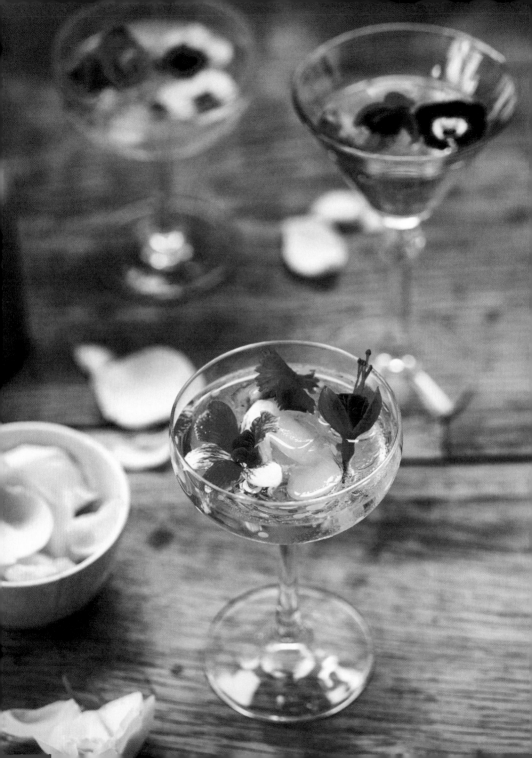

> Dry out elderflowers, store in a jar and add to your herbal tea mixes. They are great for preventing coughs and colds.

Elderflower fizz

Elderflowers remind me of my time living in the Cotswolds. When they were in season I would pick them and use them for everything. They smell so pretty. They make a wonderful edible bouquet for presents, too. This fermented elderflower concoction is delicious on its own or with a splash of soda water.

MAKES 2 LITRES

8 large heads fresh or dried elderflower

2 litres water

2 lemons, sliced

400g sugar

1 tablespoon apple cider vinegar

sterilised glass bottle

Place all the ingredients in a large ceramic bowl. Stir together until the sugar has dissolved. Cover with a clean tea towel and place in a warm (not too hot), dry place for 7–14 days.

Taste after a week and if you like the flavour you can stop fermentation at any time by transferring to a sterilised glass bottle and storing in the fridge. This will last for up to 2 weeks.

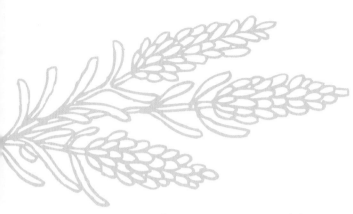

Poppy sleepy milk

Poppies have long been a symbol of sleep, peace and... death(!). I can promise you this sleepy tea will not kill you, but it will give you a dreamy sleep, as poppies in tiny doses are a sedative. The addition of hops makes for a perfect after-dinner, before-bedtime drink, as hops also help to aid rest.

SERVES 2

500ml whole milk or nut milk
1½ teaspoons finely chopped (peeled) fresh turmeric root or ground turmeric
pinch of black pepper
1½ teaspoons ground poppy seeds
1 cinnamon stick
1 teaspoon vanilla extract
1 teaspoon dried hops
2 teaspoons raw honey
2 sprigs of dried culinary lavender, to serve

Place everything, except the honey and lavender sprigs, in a saucepan and bring to a simmer over a low heat. Simmer for 5 minutes, then turn off the heat and leave the mixture to cool for a minute. Stir in the honey to dissolve. Strain into mugs or cups and serve each with a sprig of lavender.

Spiced rose lassi

I need to have as much natural yogurt in my diet as possible to protect my gut as it's a little on the leaky side. I find it hard to just eat it straight up all the time so love to mix it up with other good-for-me spices. This rose lassi is absolutely gorgeous. Serve it really chilled for a perfect Sunday brunch.

SERVES 4

375g natural yogurt
3 tablespoons raw honey
4 teaspoons rose water, or to taste
¼ teaspoon ground cardamom
pinch of ground cinnamon
pinch of salt
a little pink food colouring gel (optional)
fresh rose petals, unsprayed, to garnish

Place everything, except the rose petals, in a blender with 60ml water and blitz until smooth. Taste and add more rose water, if needed. Pour into chilled glasses to serve. Garnish with rose petals.

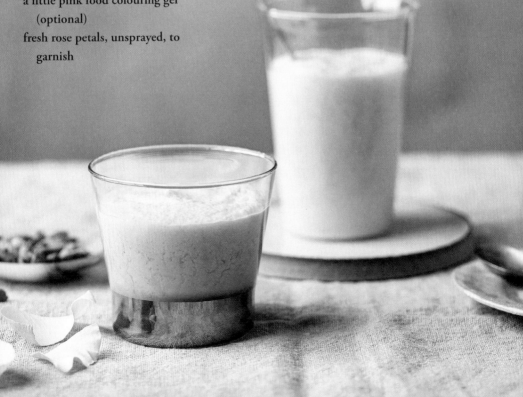

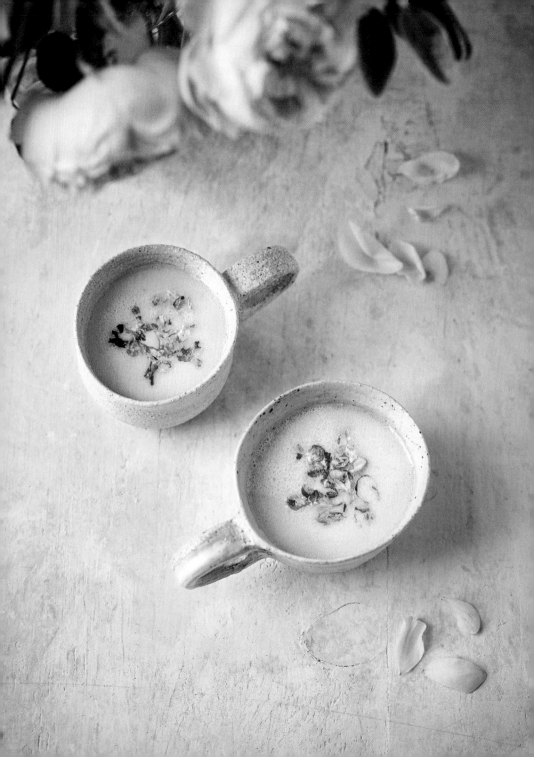

Rose and turmeric latte

Turmeric has been widely researched and the compound curcumin is believed to provide a plethora of health benefits. It also has an extremely safe profile so is a wonderful addition to anyone's daily diet. Rose and turmeric are a match made in heaven in this latte.

SERVES 1

250ml almond or coconut milk

3.5cm fresh turmeric root, peeled and roughly chopped

seeds from 2 cardamom pods, crushed

pinch of freshly ground black pepper

1–2 tablespoons rose water

1 teaspoon coconut oil

1 teaspoon raw honey or maple syrup, to taste

dried rose petals, to garnish

Place the almond or coconut milk in a blender with the turmeric, cardamom, pepper, rose water and coconut oil. Blend to combine. Warm in a small saucepan to a light simmer if drinking warm. Turn off the heat and sweeten with honey or maple syrup to taste. Drink cold or warm, garnished with rose petals.

If you want to increase the quantities and make a large batch to drink throughout the week, it will keep in a covered jug in the fridge for 4–5 days.

Floral chai

I have forever loved chai and always wanted to create my own perfect flowery version, so I think this is wonderful. Apart from tasting gorgeous, the dry ingredients make a wonderful gift in a little jar with instructions on a label and a pretty ribbon.

SERVES 4

1 teaspoon dried chamomile flowers
1 teaspoon dried rose petals
1 teaspoon dried violets
½ teaspoon dried culinary lavender
1 teaspoon cardamom seeds
3 cloves
pinch of ground white pepper
1 teaspoon ground cinnamon
1 star anise
4 teaspoons black tea
1 vanilla pod, split lengthways and seeds scraped out
600ml whole milk or nut milk
2 tablespoons honey
1 tablespoon rose water

You can either make the tea to store in a clean jar or for gifts by blending together all of the dried ingredients with the seeds of the vanilla pod until finely ground and combined. Just mix and keep in a sterilised jar in a cool, dark place for up to 3 months.

When you are ready to drink, simply add the tea mixture to the milk in a saucepan and bring to a simmer over a low–medium heat. Simmer for 5 minutes, then strain into mugs, stir in the honey and rose water and serve.

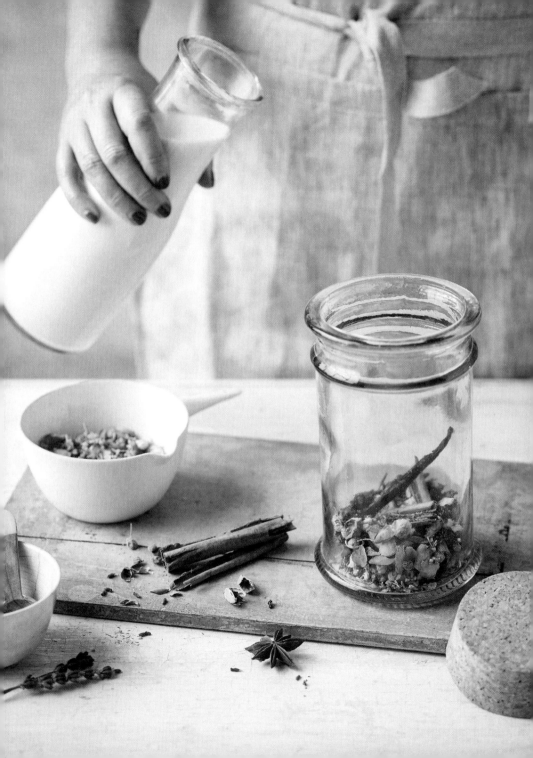

Chapter Two

desserts & baking

Floral mess

The perfect excuse to make a creative mess. Eton mess reminds me of summer and this recipe is so adaptable. Try any of the petal powders from page 50 for different colours in the mess. You could even do the meringue in one colour and the cream in another. Have fun!

SERVES 4–6

3 large free-range egg whites

175g caster sugar

2 teaspoons hibiscus powder (use more for a brighter colour)

500ml double cream

2 tablespoons icing sugar, or to taste

500g fresh berries (such as raspberries, strawberries, blueberries or mulberries)

2 handfuls of fresh edible flowers

Preheat the oven to 130°C/gas mark 1. Line a baking tray with baking paper and set aside.

Whisk the egg whites in a clean, dry stainless steel bowl until soft peaks form. You can do this with a stand mixer, if you prefer. Add the caster sugar, a spoonful at a time, and keep whisking until dissolved. Gently fold through half the hibiscus powder.

Spoon the meringue into four large mounds on the lined baking tray and bake on the middle shelf of the oven for 1 hour. Turn off the oven and leave the meringues in there until completely cold.

In a mixing bowl, whip the cream with the icing sugar and the remaining hibiscus powder until thick. Gently fold in the berries. Smash up the meringues and place them in serving bowls, then spoon over the berry cream, dividing it evenly. Decorate with the edible flowers and serve.

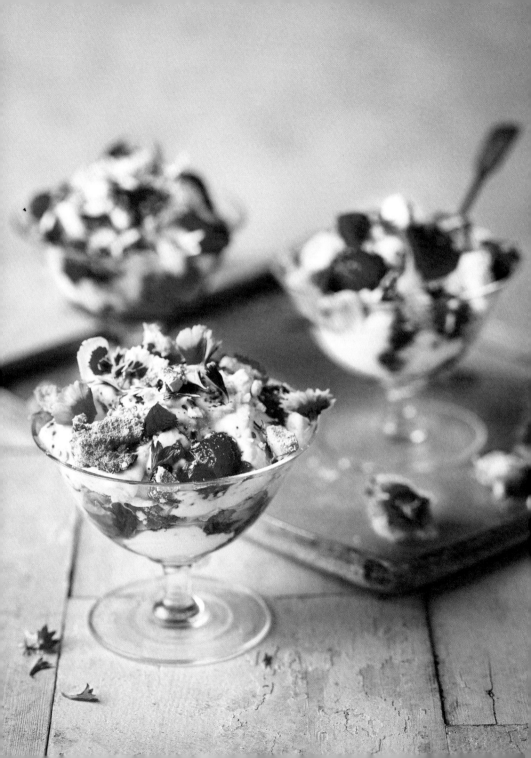

Chilli & rose chocolate tart

Once you perfect this recipe, the flower combinations are endless. You just need to infuse the cream with your choice of aromats and flowers.

SERVES 6–8

for the pastry

150g butter, softened, plus extra for greasing

100g coconut sugar

200g raw cacao powder

2 teaspoons honey

250g plain flour, plus extra for dusting

pinch of salt

for the filling

2 medium or hot fresh red chillies, roughly chopped

1 tablespoon rosewater

1 tablespoon dried rose petals

600ml double cream

400g good-quality dark chocolate

candied flowers or dried/fresh unsprayed rose petals

For the pastry, cream the butter and sugar together until light and fluffy, then add the cacao and honey and beat for a minute more. Add the flour and salt and stir. Wrap in greaseproof paper and chill in the fridge for 1 hour. Preheat your oven to 200°C/gas mark 6. Meanwhile, poach the chillies in the cream with the rosewater and rose petals over a low heat for about 20 minutes – taste as you go to get the right flavour. Scoop out the chillies, squeeze, then discard.

Lightly grease a 23cm flan dish. Roll out the pastry and use it to line the prepared dish. Prick the pastry case all over with a fork, then line with greaseproof paper and fill with a layer of baking beans. Bake for 20 minutes, then remove the paper and beans and bake for a further 5 minutes until fully cooked and golden brown. Leave to cool completely.

Break up the chocolate and add to the warm chilli cream, then gently whisk until it forms a smooth ganache. Transfer to the fridge to cool and thicken.

Once cool, spoon the ganache into the pastry case and spread evenly, then chill for at least 1 hour before serving. Decorate with candied flowers or rose petals just before serving.

Rose, carob & coconut granola

This is packed full of health, flavour and wake-me-up aromas. Perfect for your breakfast or as an afternoon pick-me-up snack on its own by the handful. It also makes a wonderful little gift in a pretty jar with some ribbon. The roses can be replaced with any dried edible flower.

MAKES 10 SERVINGS

500g coconut flakes, unsweetened
220g chopped mixed nuts
150g pumpkin seeds
100g sunflower seeds
100g raw cacao nibs
50g dried rose petals
3 tablespoons chia seeds
1 tablespoon raw cacao powder
1 teaspoon carob powder
1 teaspoon ground cinnamon
100–125g coconut oil, melted (the more you use, the chewier your granola will be – use less if you prefer it crunchier)
3 tablespoons maple syrup

Preheat the oven to 150°C/gas mark 2. Line two baking trays with greaseproof paper and set aside.

Put all the dry ingredients into a large bowl and mix thoroughly. Stir in the melted coconut oil and maple syrup a little at a time and mix well. You don't want the mix to be soggy, just coated, or the end result won't be crispy. Spread the mixture out on the lined baking trays, trying to space it all evenly in a single layer. Bake for 10–15 minutes, or until golden brown. Stir or shake the trays a few times during the cooking time.

Remove from the oven and leave to cool completely. Once cool, tip the granola into an airtight jar and use within two weeks. This granola contains oil, which may fall to the bottom of the jar or solidify during storage. Don't worry if this happens – just mix it back in.

Flower granitas four ways

Granitas are a little underrated. They are really very simple to make, they allow for many a combination and are always a perfect dinner party palate cleanser to impress your guests. They are also worth considering as a vegan alternative to ice creams. Play around with combinations and flavours using a basic sugar syrup and juice mix or infused sugar syrup. Use what's in season for a really cheap dinner party dazzler.

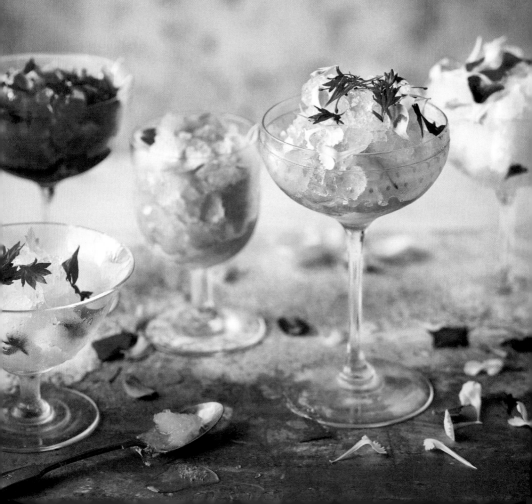

Honeysuckle & Hibiscus

SERVES 4–6

**3 handfuls fresh honeysuckle
flowers, plus extra to decorate**
**1 tablespoon dried whole hibiscus
flowers**
1 cinnamon stick, crushed
225g caster sugar
1 teaspoon lemon juice

Place the honeysuckle and hibiscus flowers and cinnamon in a heatproof bowl, then pour over 700ml water. Cover with a tea towel and leave for 48 hours at room temperature.

Strain into a clean bowl, discarding the flowers and cinnamon, and set aside.

Make a sugar syrup by combining 250ml water and the sugar in a pan, then heat gently for 2 minutes or so, stirring occasionally, until the sugar dissolves. Remove from the heat and stir through the lemon juice and the flower-infused water.

Pour into a deep baking tray or shallow freezerproof dish and put in the freezer for 1 hour. Using a fork, scrape the iced mixture, stirring the crystals from around the edges into the centre and mashing well. Return to the freezer and repeat the process three more times every hour or so until the mixture is completely frozen (it should be the texture of snow).

Fork the granita up roughly to serve and serve in glasses or bowls, decorated with fresh honeysuckle blooms.

Violet & Mint

SERVES 4–6

4 handfuls fresh violets
480ml boiling water
500g caster sugar
1 teaspoon lemon juice
small handful of fresh mint

Place the violets in a heatproof bowl, then pour over the boiling water. Cover with a tea towel and leave overnight at room temperature.

The next day, strain through a sieve into a saucepan, squishing the violets as you go. Stir in the sugar and heat slowly until very gently simmering, stirring. Don't boil, just heat until the sugar dissolves. Turn off the heat and add the lemon juice if you want purple liquid – without it will stay blue. Set aside to cool.

Now pick off and reserve the mint flowers, then pick and finely chop the mint leaves. Once the syrup is completely cool, add the chopped mint.

Pour into a deep baking tray or shallow freezerproof dish and follow the instructions for freezing on page 35. Fork the granita up roughly and serve in glasses or bowls, decorated with fresh violets and the reserved mint flowers.

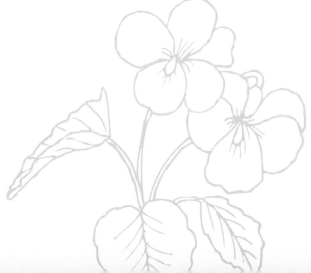

Orange Blossom, Watermelon & Carnation

SERVES 4–6

225g caster sugar

1 handful fresh carnation petals, unsprayed, plus extra blooms to decorate

2 tablespoons orange blossom water

450g prepared watermelon, puréed and strained to make 500ml

In a large saucepan, bring the sugar and 240ml water to the boil over a medium–high heat, stirring to dissolve the sugar. Reduce the heat, then simmer for about 2 minutes, stirring occasionally. Remove from the heat and add the carnation petals. Leave to cool, then add the orange blossom water and strain through a sieve. Mix the syrup and watermelon juice together. Pour into a deep baking tray or shallow freezerproof dish and follow the instructions for freezing on page 35. Fork the granita up roughly and serve decorated with fresh carnation blooms.

Rose, Carnation & Basil

SERVES 4–6

200g fresh rose petals, unsprayed and perfumed, plus extra to decorate

200g fresh carnation petals, unsprayed

500g caster sugar

2 sprigs of basil, leaves picked and stalks roughly chopped, plus extra sprigs to decorate

zest and juice of 1 lemon

1–2 tablespoons rose water, to taste

Place the rose and carnation petals in a bowl with the sugar and basil, stir gently to combine, then cover with a tea towel. Leave overnight.

The next day, strain through a sieve into a saucepan, add 750ml water and stir until the sugar dissolves. Bring to the boil over a high heat, then reduce the heat and simmer for a few minutes. Turn off the heat, then stir in the lemon zest and juice and the rose water.

Pour into a deep baking tray or shallow freezerproof dish and follow the instructions for freezing on page 35. Fork the granita up roughly and serve in glasses or bowls, decorated with fresh rose petals and basil sprigs.

Elderflower jelly

This is so very pretty and delicate. If you don't have elderflower cordial you can actually use any type of cordial so long as you stick to the measurements. This has a very grown-up feel to it and would be wonderful with the addition of berries or fresh mint leaves.

SERVES 4

100g caster sugar
4 gelatine leaves
100ml elderflower cordial
fresh edible flowers or petals,
   to decorate

Put the sugar in a pan with 400ml water and bring to the boil, stirring so the sugar dissolves. Remove from the heat.

Meanwhile, soak the gelatine leaves in cold water for a few minutes to soften. Gently squeeze the excess water from the gelatine, then add to the hot syrup and stir until dissolved. Add the cordial to the syrup and stir.

Pour into 4 individual clear glasses, jars or little bowls and leave to set in the fridge overnight. Serve in the bowls or turned out onto plates, decorated with edible flowers or petals on the top.

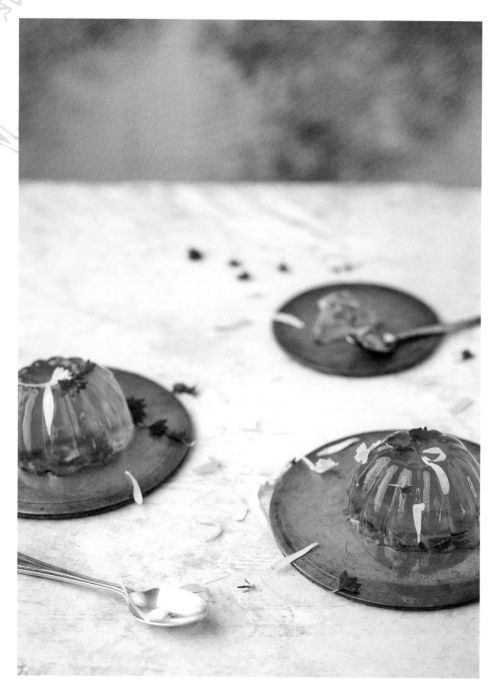

Flower fritters

These can easily be made savoury by not adding the icing sugar or food colouring and spicing the seasoning with whatever you like really. They make a gorgeous dessert dusted with pastel-coloured icing sugar.

SERVES 2–4

65g icing sugar
natural pink colouring
    (preferably gel)
vegetable oil, for deep-frying
10–15 wild fennel or elderflower
    heads with about 5cm stems
    (you could use any edible
    flowers)

for the batter

55g rice flour
55g plain flour
½ teaspoon baking powder
pinch of salt
1 free-range egg
300ml soda water, chilled

Add all of the batter ingredients to a bowl and mix until combined. It is important not to overmix and don't worry if it is not super smooth. Set aside.

Mix the icing sugar with some pink food colouring gel using your fingers until evenly coloured. Set aside.

Pour enough vegetable oil into a deep saucepan to fill it one-third full. Heat over a medium–high heat until a little drop of batter sizzles immediately when dropped in.

Now dip the heads of the flowers into the batter to coat and shake off any excess. Holding the stem, place each into the hot oil and fry for 1–2 minutes, or until golden brown. They are really delicate so don't need to cook for long at all. Don't overcrowd the pan and just deep-fry a few at a time.

Once cooked, remove using a slotted spoon and place on kitchen paper to remove excess oil. Using a sieve or sifter, dust with the pink icing sugar, then serve.

Cornflower, chamomile & lemon shortbread

My family all fight over shortbread at Christmas time. My nan spends weeks baking batches for all the family (28 of us) and puts them into recycled tins and jars. It's a bit of a contentious issue because if someone gets a bigger tin or jar, the fights begin immediately. Nan, this recipe is for you.

MAKES 10–12

75g caster sugar
2 teaspoons lemon zest, plus extra
    for sprinkling
125g butter, softened
150g plain flour
pinch of salt
2 teaspoons dried blue or
    pink cornflowers
1 teaspoon chamomile
    flower powder

Line a large baking tray with greaseproof paper. Put the sugar, lemon zest and butter in a bowl and mix together with an electric mixer until light and fluffy. Add the flour, salt and cornflower and chamomile powders and mix on low until just combined. Put the mix onto the lined baking tray in a loose ball, then refrigerate for 10 minutes.

Remove from the fridge and roll the shortbread into a log shape of about 20cm. Wrap in greaseproof paper and chill in the fridge for an hour.

Preheat the oven to 180°C/gas mark 4. Unwrap the shortbread and slice it into 2cm thick rounds. Place the rounds on the lined baking tray, leaving space in between each one. Sprinkle with some extra lemon zest.

Bake for 15–18 minutes, or until golden brown on the edges. Cool on the tray for a few minutes, then transfer to a wire rack and leave to cool completely. Store in an airtight container (or jar/tin) for up to a week, ensuring you don't give one family member more than the other.

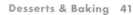

Lavender & orange cheesecake

This is my mum's favourite dessert that I make. It's really not very fancy and is so easy to make. As the filling contains no gelatine, this cheesecake has a very soft set; if you prefer a firmer set, use 400g cream cheese and 150ml double cream.

SERVES 6–8

for the base

butter, for greasing

100g ginger nut biscuits, crushed

150g butternut snap cookies or digestives, crushed

zest of ½ an orange (use the other half for the topping)

1 teaspoon culinary lavender

80g butter

for the topping

340g cream cheese, softened

200ml double cream

zest and juice of ½ an orange

115g unrefined caster sugar

2 tablespoons orange blossom water

fresh edible flowers, to decorate

For the base, lightly grease a 23cm springform tin with butter. Mix together the crushed buscuits and stir in the orange zest and lavender.

Melt the butter in a small saucepan and then mix it evenly into the crumbs. Press the crumb mixture firmly over the base of the greased tin. Put the tin in the fridge to set while you make the topping.

In a mixing bowl, beat the cream cheese with an electric mixer just to loosen it until it is the consistency of thickened cream. This should take no longer than 45–60 seconds.

In a separate bowl, whip the cream until thick. Gently fold the whipped cream into the cream cheese. Add the orange zest and juice, sugar and orange blossom water and fold together until the mixture resembles thick cream.

Spread the topping evenly over the biscuit base using a spatula or knife. Return to the fridge and leave to set for an hour or so, then decorate with the edible flowers just before serving.

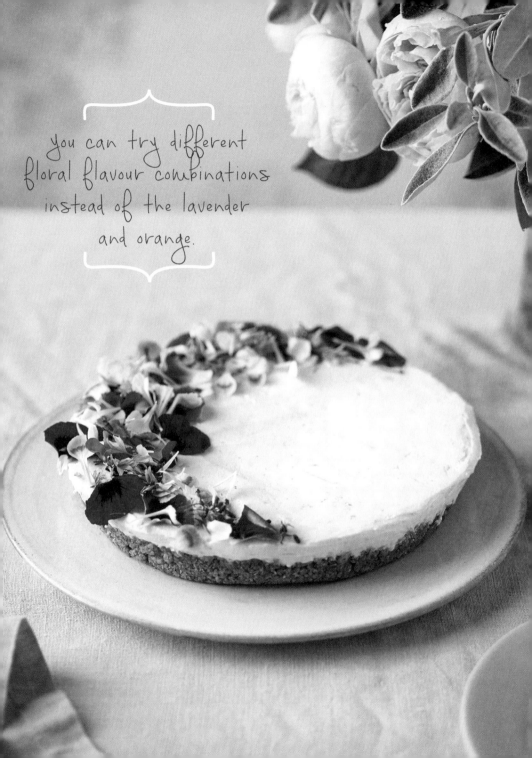

you can try different floral flavour combinations instead of the lavender and orange.

Strawberry, hibiscus & peony swiss roll

This is a very lady-like Swiss Roll and is filled with delicious jam and hibiscus-scented cream. What a gorgeous birthday cake this makes!

SERVES 4

4 free-range eggs

115g caster sugar

50g butter, melted, plus extra for greasing

130g self-raising flour, sifted

500ml double cream

3 tablespoons icing sugar

1 teaspoon hibiscus powder

320g strawberry jam

fresh peonies, to decorate

Preheat the oven to 180°C/gas mark 4. Grease and line a Swiss roll tin (about 30 x 21cm).

In a bowl, whisk the eggs and caster sugar together. Add the melted butter and whisk it in, then gently fold in the sifted flour. Pour into the prepared tin and even out. Bake for 10 minutes, until lightly browned.

Line your work surface with a sheet of baking paper bigger than the sponge. Turn the sponge out of the tin onto the paper, then carefully peel the lining paper off the base of the sponge. Transfer to a wire rack (still on the paper) and leave to cool completely.

Using an electric mixer, whip the cream with the icing sugar until thick. Divide it into two bowls and add the hibiscus powder to one so it turns pink.

Spread the inside of the cake with a thick layer of jam and then a layer of the white cream. Score the sponge lightly about 2.5cm in from one short end. Roll it up carefully using the paper to help you, then neaten up the ends with a knife. To finish, spread a thick layer of the pink hibiscus cream over the outside of the cake and scatter peonies over the top.

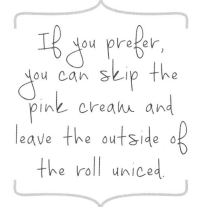

If you prefer, you can skip the pink cream and leave the outside of the roll uniced.

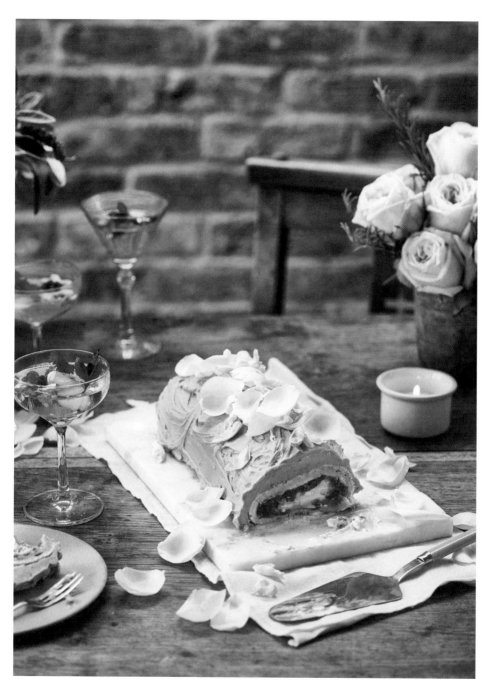

Geranium sherbet

I have to admit my love affair with geraniums is quite new. I only recently found out they were edible. Before then, I snubbed them. Bad me. The petals are exquisite in colour and the leaves edible too. Add both the petals and leaves to salads too for a lemony and colourful kick.

SERVES 4

55g caster sugar

540ml buttermilk

2 large handfuls of fresh geranium petals, plus a few leaves

120ml agave syrup/nectar

1 teaspoon rose water, plus extra to serve

to decorate

coarsely chopped roasted pistachios

fresh geranium flower petals

Place the sugar in a small saucepan with 60ml of the buttermilk and the geranium petals and leaves. Cook over a medium heat, stirring, until the sugar has completely dissolved. Pour into a heatproof bowl, then add the remaining buttermilk. Stir in the agave syrup/nectar and rose water. Leave to infuse in the fridge for a couple of hours.

Pour into an ice-cream maker and churn according to the manufacturer's instructions.

Once it's ready, line a small (20cm) loaf tin with clingfilm, spoon the sherbet mixture into the tin, then cover with clingfilm and freeze for at least 1 hour before serving, and for up to a week.

To serve, scoop the sherbet into bowls. Decorate each portion with a few drops of rose water, some chopped pistachios and a few flower petals.

Jasmine & green tea ice cream

This is the purest form of ice cream, and the joy of it is that you don't need an ice-cream maker, nor do you need to churn it in any way. You can easily try different types of tea and dried flowers by infusing the cream in the same way, then just make and freeze.

SERVES 1–2

250ml double cream
1 teaspoon green tea
1 teaspoon jasmine tea (flowers)
3 tablespoons runny honey
3 free-range egg yolks
seeds scraped from ½ vanilla pod
**   or 1 teaspoon vanilla extract**
fresh jasmine flowers, to decorate

In a saucepan, gently heat the cream with the two teas for a couple of minutes. Remove from the heat and pour into a container. Once cool, cover and leave in the fridge overnight to infuse.

The next day, strain the cream.

Heat the honey in a small saucepan until just warmed. Put the egg yolks in a mixing bowl and whisk in the warm honey. Whisk in the cream and vanilla until thick. Pour into a freezerproof serving dish. Freeze for 2–3 hours, or until firm. Serve decorated with fresh jasmine flowers.

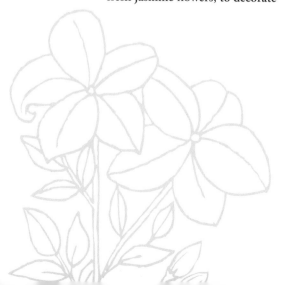

Chapter Three
sweets

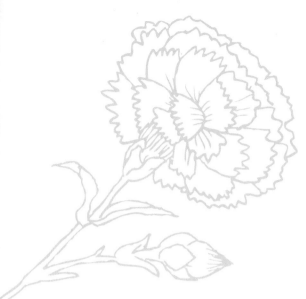

Petal powders

Use the petals of any dried edible flower for this recipe, and ensure they are crispy dry. These are great to use for any desserts that need a kick of colour.

GREAT PETALS TO USE ARE:

calendula

carnations

chamomile

cornflowers

hibiscus

marigolds

roses

violets

Place the dried petals in small batches into a spice grinder and blitz until you get a fine powder. Store in airtight containers and use for all sorts of things.

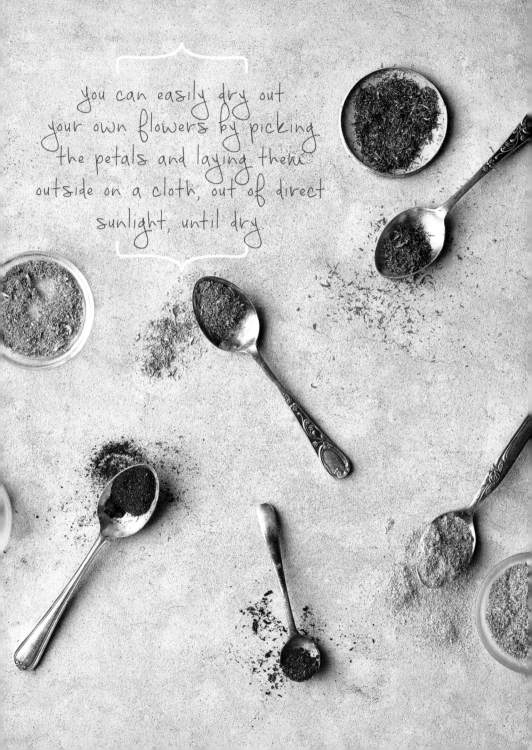

You can easily dry out
your own flowers by picking
the petals and laying them
outside on a cloth, out of direct
sunlight, until dry

Crystallised petals & flowers

These make the perfect addition to any cake or are ideal for a wonderful wedding bomboniere, hen do or grown-up party bag. You can pretty much crystallise most petals, just play around with them until you find your favourites.

MAKES ABOUT 100G

2 large handfuls of fresh rose petals, unsprayed
2 handfuls of small or 1 handful of large edible flowers
110–225g caster sugar
3 free-range egg whites

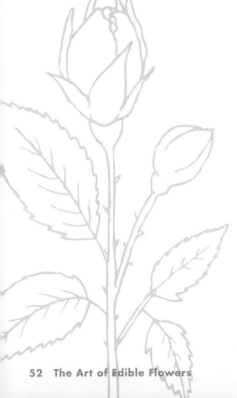

Line two baking trays with greaseproof paper and set aside.

Remove and shake out any little critters from the petals and flowers. You can rinse them but will then need to wait until they are thoroughly dried before using. Cut the head of the rose from the stem of the flower. Carefully hold the bud and begin to pull off the petals from the middle and place aside.

Pour the sugar into a small bowl. Lightly whisk the egg whites in another small bowl until frothy. Now get a production line going.

Using a pastry brush, lightly brush each rose petal front and back with egg white. Dip into the sugar, evenly coating each side of the petal, then place it onto a lined baking tray. Repeat with the remainder of the rose petals and flowers. Once they are all coated, leave them somewhere warm but not humid overnight to dry. They will be ready when they are hard enough to eat like sweets.

Store in an airtight container for up to a week, taking care to keep the layers separate with baking paper.

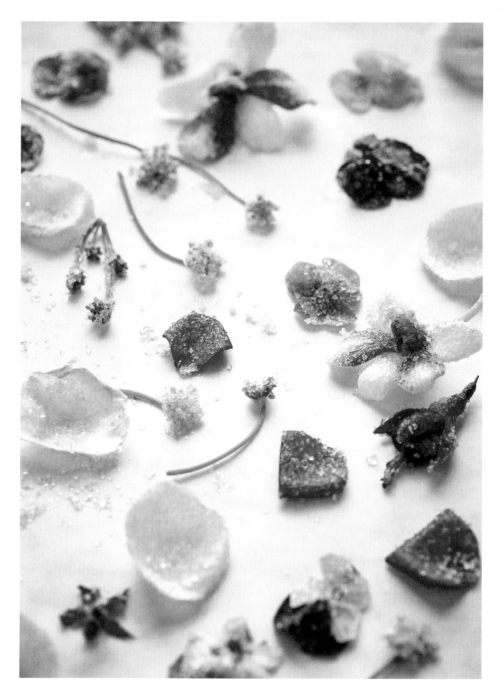

Rose marshmallows coated in lavender chocolate

Marshmallows aren't just for kids or bonfires. They are for all the time and for everyone! Especially these ones.

MAKES 20

olive oil spray, for greasing
4½ teaspoons powdered gelatine
165g caster sugar
125ml glucose syrup
¼ teaspoon salt
2 teaspoons rose water
pink food colouring gel
200g good-quality dark chocolate
2 teaspoons culinary lavender or a
   few drops of lavender oil

to decorate

fresh rose petals and lavender
   flowers, unsprayed, or dried

Lightly coat a small shallow baking tin with olive oil spray. In a small bowl, whisk together the gelatine and 60ml water, then leave it to sit for 5 minutes.

Make a syrup by placing the sugar, 60ml of the glucose syrup, the salt and 120ml water into a medium saucepan over a high heat. Bring to the boil, stir until the sugar has dissolved, then continue boiling, stirring, until the temperature reaches 115°C on a thermometer.

Put the remaining glucose syrup into the bowl of your stand mixer. Microwave the gelatine mix on high until melted, about 30 seconds, stirring once or twice. Pour into the stand mixer bowl, then turn the mixer on to low and keep it running. Slowly pour the syrup into the mixer bowl, whisking continuously. Increase the speed to medium and whisk for 5 minutes, then increase to medium–high for another 5 minutes. Add the rose water and food colouring to the desired colour, then increase to the highest speed and whisk until fluffy.

Pour the mixture into the greased baking tin, banging the tray on the worktop to spread evenly and smoothing the surface with a palette knife. Leave in a cool, dry place for about 6 hours to set.

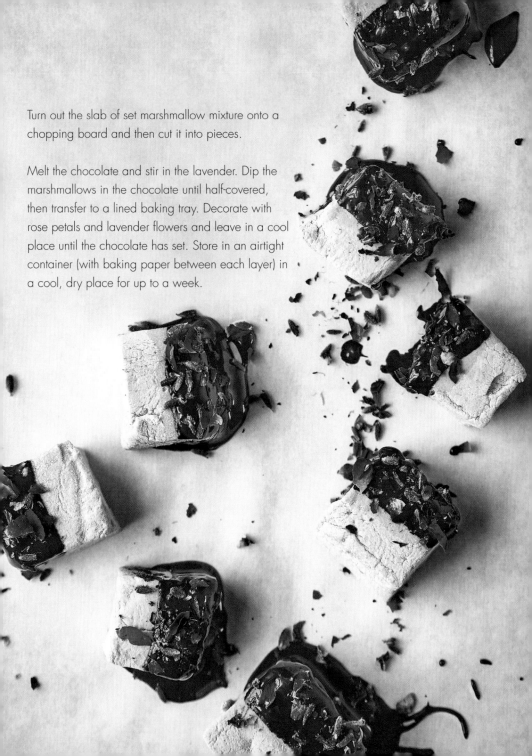

Turn out the slab of set marshmallow mixture onto a chopping board and then cut it into pieces.

Melt the chocolate and stir in the lavender. Dip the marshmallows in the chocolate until half-covered, then transfer to a lined baking tray. Decorate with rose petals and lavender flowers and leave in a cool place until the chocolate has set. Store in an airtight container (with baking paper between each layer) in a cool, dry place for up to a week.

Orange blossom truffles

These are a cross between a ganache-like truffle and a bliss ball. They kind of feel healthy but decadent too.

MAKES 10–12

75g dried stoned dates
75g dried stoned prunes
75g dried apricots
2 tablespoons orange blossom
water
1 teaspoon ground cinnamon
zest of 1 orange
pinch of sea salt
100g good-quality dark chocolate
(at least 70 per cent cocoa solids)
25g butter, diced
125g ground almonds
Rose Petal and Calendula Petal
Powders (see page 50)

Roughly chop the dates, prunes and apricots and tip into a bowl. Cover them with room temperature water, then cover with a tea towel and leave to soak for 2 hours.

Drain the soaked fruit and then add to a food-processor with the orange blossom water, cinnamon, orange zest and sea salt. Pulse, stopping to stir everything every now and then, until you have a smooth paste.

Break the chocolate into pieces and melt with the butter in a heatproof bowl over a saucepan of barely simmering water (or in a double boiler). Take the melted chocolate mix off the heat. Add the fruit mixture and ground almonds and stir well. Chill in the fridge for 1 hour.

Line a baking tray with baking paper. Spoon the petal powders onto separate plates. Scoop a heaped teaspoonful of the chocolate truffle mixture and roll it into a ball, then roll in the petal powders. Place each coated truffle on the lined baking tray. Repeat until you've used up all the truffle mixture.

Refrigerate the truffles for a few hours to firm them up. Transfer to an airtight container, separating the layers with baking paper. They will keep for up to 5 days in the fridge.

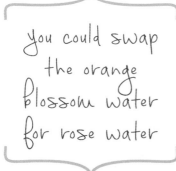

You could swap the orange blossom water for rose water

Rosehip & apple fruit leather

This recipe is from my dear friend and stylist on this book series, Rachel. She was playing about with fruit leathers the entire time we were shooting and we fell in love with this fragrant and delicate combination.

SERVES 8–10

400g apples (cooking apples are fine)
4 tablespoons fresh rosehips
50g raw honey
splash of rose water
pinch of ground cinnamon

Preheat the oven to 110°C/gas mark ¼ and line a baking tray with greaseproof paper.

Peel and core the apples, then dice them. Cook the apples by simmering in a small pan of water for about 10 minutes until they are just soft but not soggy. At the same time, put the rosehips in a small pan, cover with a small amount of water and simmer until soft too, about 10–15 minutes.

Once cooked, squeeze the rosehips through a piece of muslin into a food-processor and then add the apples too. Add the honey, rose water and cinnamon and process until smooth.

Spoon the mixture into small paper-thin circles on the lined baking tray, then bake for an hour, or until they are bendy (or, if you prefer them crisp, a little longer). Remove from the oven and leave to cool completely on the baking tray, then carefully peel each leather off the paper. Store in an airtight container, with baking paper between each layer, for up to a week.

Almond and flower fudge

I think fudge fits into the love or hate category. It is sweet, and can be sickly. This one is indeed sweet, but luckily not sickly. The addition of nuts for texture and flowers for colour make an unusual and tasty sweet treat.

MAKES 20 PIECES

200g coconut oil
200g icing sugar
100g almonds, chopped
2 tablespoons dried cornflowers
or 2 teaspoons petal powder
(page 50)

Line a shallow tin measuring about 15–20cm square with baking paper.

Place the coconut oil and icing sugar in a bowl and use a stick blender to blend until emulsified. Stir in the nuts and about half of the flowers or powder.

Transfer this mixture to the tin and spread it out evenly, smoothing the surface. Sprinkle the remaining flowers on top and place in the fridge for a couple of hours until set.

Slice into small pieces to serve. Store in the fridge and eat within 2 weeks.

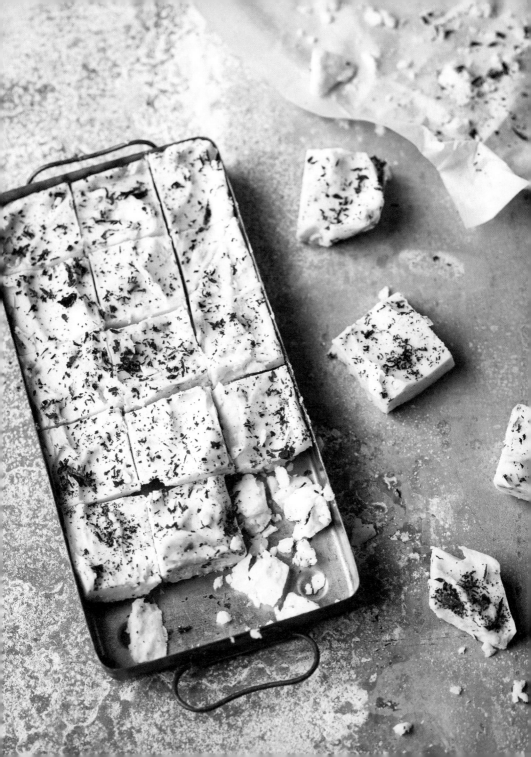

Chapter Four
savoury

Try these sprinkled with garlic salt, paprika and sea salt or dried onion. The combinations are endless.

Salt & vinegar leaf crisps

These are simply ace. A little like kale crisps but with more texture. Try this recipe with any edible leaves and different kinds of salt and spice combinations.

SERVES 2–4

60ml apple cider vinegar
large pinch of sea salt
2 handfuls of edible flower leaves,
such as fig, blackcurrant or vine
1 teaspoon chilli flakes (optional)

spray bottle

Preheat the oven to 160°C/gas mark 3. Line a baking tray with greaseproof paper.

Shake the vinegar and salt together in a spray bottle and then spray the flower leaves lightly all over. Spread the leaves out on the lined baking tray in a single layer. Sprinkle with chilli flakes for an extra kick.

Bake for about 10 minutes, or until crisp. Remove from the oven and leave to cool completely on the baking tray. Store in an airtight container – they will keep for a few days.

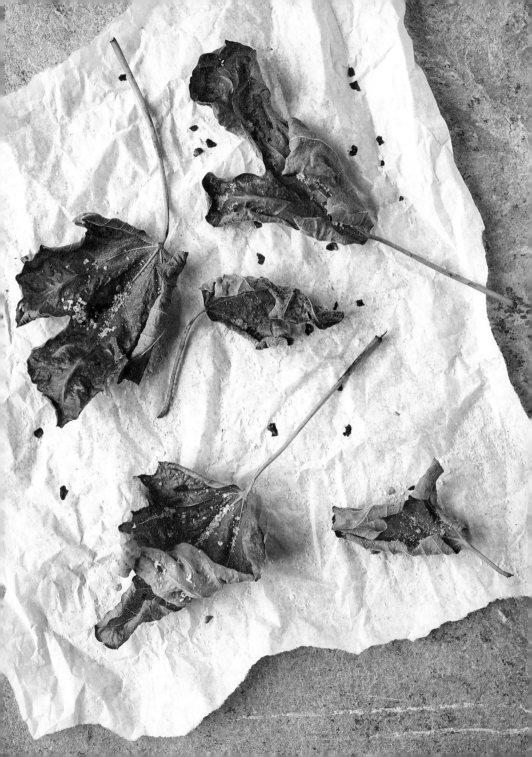

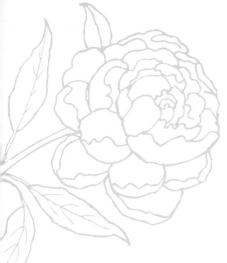

Pickled peony & primrose petals

Whoever would have thought it? But these pickled petals make a wonderful addition to a cheese board, in a toastie or scattered through a salad. They will lose their colour in the jar but will hold their flavour for months.

MAKES 2 X 250ML JARS

480ml apple cider vinegar (or use raw or kombucha vinegar)

8 tablespoons raw honey

1 tablespoon salt

8 cloves

1 cinnamon stick

2 star anise

1 slice of orange peel

2 handfuls fresh primrose petals, unsprayed

2 handfuls fresh peony petals, unsprayed (or you can just use unsprayed and perfumed rose petals in place of both types of petals)

2 sterilised 250ml jars

Place all the ingredients, except the petals, in a saucepan and bring to the boil, stirring once or twice. Remove from the heat and leave to cool for 10 minutes, then pour over the mixed petals in a heatproof bowl or jug.

Transfer into hot, sterilised jars, then seal and leave to cool. Label and store in a cool, dark place for a month before eating. These are delicious in salads – just remove some petals from the jar with a little of the liquid and toss through the salad. The pickling liquid has lots of great flavour too. Refrigerate after opening.

Nasturtium capers

I love capers very much, so when I realised that you could pickle nasturtium pods and they had the same texture and little zing as capers do, I was very excited. Use these delicious little pickles in just about everything.

MAKES 4 X 250ML JARS

800g fresh nasturtium pods, picked when still green

50g salt

450ml water

220g white granulated sugar

500ml apple cider vinegar

250ml white wine vinegar

2 teaspoons yellow mustard seeds

1 teaspoon black mustard seeds

1 teaspoon celery seeds

1 blade of mace or ½ teaspoon grated nutmeg

1 teaspoon fennel seeds

4 sterilised 250ml jars

Combine the nasturtium pods, salt and water in a bowl, cover with a tea towel and leave overnight at room temperature.

The next day, drain the pods and place in a heatproof bowl. Set aside.

In a medium saucepan, combine all the remaining ingredients and bring to the boil, stirring initially to dissolve the sugar, then simmer covered for 20 minutes, stirring occasionally.

Remove from the heat, pour over the nasturtium pods and leave for a few minutes before pouring into hot, sterilised jars, then seal and leave to cool. Label and store in a cool, dark place for up to a year, and let them mature for at least a month or two before eating. Refrigerate after opening.

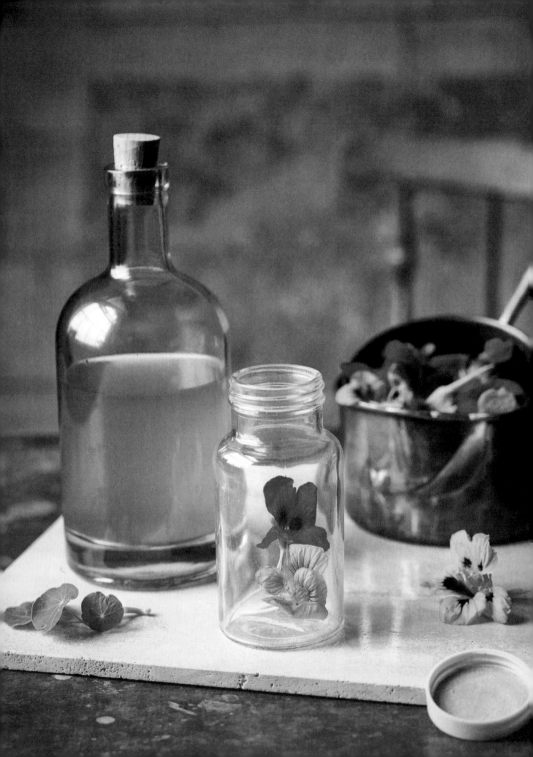

Flower & leaf vinegars

Fun to make and fun to give. These can literally be any combination you like. Pick and forage to your heart's content and make different ones for the seasons.

SUITABLE VINEGARS

apple cider

kombucha (best stored in the fridge)

malt

red wine

white wine

rice

fruit

SOME SUITABLE
FLOWERS & LEAVES
(but experiment with
your own choice too)

blackcurrant leaves

elderflowers and berries

fig leaves

**lemon verbena and lemon balm
   leaves**

nasturtium flowers

rose petals

tomato leaves (not flowers)

vine leaves

calendula

rose geranium

sterilised glass bottles

To make, use about a handful of your chosen flowers and leaves per 500ml of vinegar. Steep the fresh flowers and leaves in the vinegars (in sealed sterilised glass bottles or jars) for a few months before using as you would a normal vinegar. Bitter leaves need to be strained out after a month or so to avoid imparting too much bitter flavour. Other leaves can stay in, but I suggest refreshing them monthly.

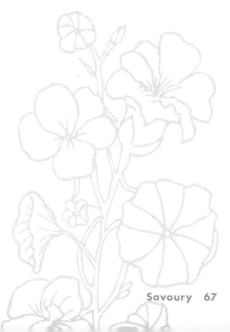

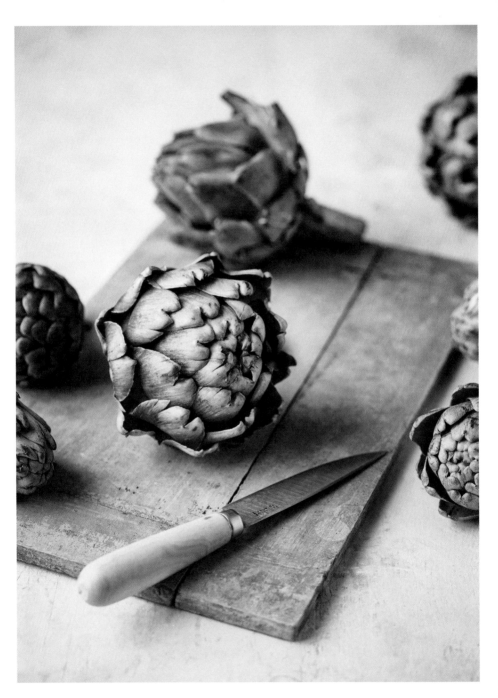

Artichokes with roasted garlic & chive flowers

This is so fabulous as a starter for a little dinner party. So much fun to eat and super garlic heavy. Artichokes are a flower and actually one of my favourites when the purple petals are out. I like to dry them out and keep them in a vase as they last for months.

SERVES 4

4 large globe artichokes
8 garlic cloves
a handful of fresh garlic flowers
a handful of fresh chive flowers
olive oil, for drizzling
juice of 2 lemons, plus extra to
serve
salt and freshly ground black
pepper

Preheat the oven to 220°C/gas mark 7. Using a sharp knife, cut off the tops (just an inch or so) of the artichokes, then using a smaller paring knife, dig out a small amount of the middle of each artichoke to make a hole. Stuff each hole with two garlic cloves and half of each of the flowers evenly. Drizzle each stuffed artichoke with olive oil and lemon juice and season with salt and pepper, ensuring you get it in between the layers.

Wrap each artichoke individually in foil, place them on a baking tray and bake for an hour, or until tender.

Serve on a plate with a sprinkle of the remaining flowers, some more oil, lemon juice and salt and pepper to taste. Eat the artichokes by removing and dipping the leaves into the roasted garlic centres.

Courgette flowers stuffed with chèvre & nasturtium capers

This is one of the easiest and most impressive dishes to make. Don't be scared of the frying part of this recipe, just test a little batter before plunging in the entire flower. You could also batter a few nasturtium flowers while you're making this, if you like.

SERVES 2–3

6 large tablespoons goat's cheese (chèvre)
2 tablespoons Nasturtium Capers (see page 65)
4–6 courgette flowers
sunflower or rapeseed oil, for frying
salt and freshly ground black pepper
runny honey, to serve

for the batter

55g rice flour
55g plain flour
½ teaspoon baking powder
pinch of salt
1 free-range egg
300ml soda water, chilled

Add all of the batter ingredients to a bowl and mix until combined. It is important not to overmix and don't worry if it's not super smooth. Set aside.

Make the stuffed flowers by mixing the goat's cheese with the capers and seasoning with salt and pepper. Using a teaspoon, carefully stuff each flower with some of the cheese mix. Twist the end of each flower to close it and enclose the filling.

Pour enough oil into a deep saucepan until it's one-third full. Heat over a medium–high heat until a little drop of batter sizzles immediately when dropped in.

Now dip the stuffed flowers into the batter to coat and shake off any excess. Place each one into the hot oil and fry for 1–2 minutes, or until golden brown. They are really delicate so don't need to cook for long at all. Don't overcrowd the pan and just deep-fry a couple at a time.

Once cooked, remove using a slotted spoon and place on kitchen paper to remove excess oil. Drizzle with honey to serve.

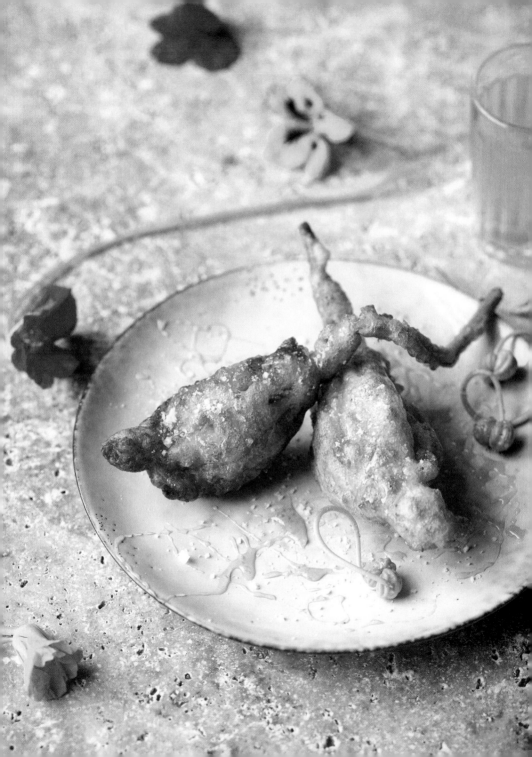

Barbecued garlic scapes with bergamot sauce

Garlic scapes contain a decent amount of protein, vitamin C and calcium. Since they're part of the garlic plant, they offer the same health benefits as the cloves, such as prevention of heart disease, high cholesterol and high blood pressure.

SERVES 6 AS A STARTER

for the sauce

1 handful fresh bergamot flowers
1 handful fresh parsley
2 garlic cloves, peeled
60ml water
240ml olive oil
zest and juice of 1 lemon
salt and freshly ground black
   pepper

for the scapes

6 small bunches of garlic scapes
   (flower buds)
2 tablespoons olive oil

For the sauce, start by very quickly blanching the bergamot flowers and parsley. Do this by pouring boiling water over them, then quickly remove them and dip them into iced water. They will turn brown when you do this, but don't fret. Now add them to a blender, along with the garlic and water, and blitz until smooth, seasoning with salt and pepper. Keeping your blender running on low, very slowly drizzle in the olive oil until everything is combined.

Transfer the sauce to a small pan and heat gently over a low heat, stirring occasionally, until hot. Whisk through the lemon juice just before serving.

Meanwhile, for the scapes, preheat a griddle pan on the hob until hot or preheat your barbecue. Season your scapes with the olive oil and some salt and pepper and then grill on the griddle pan or over the barbecue for about 5 minutes until they begin to go golden brown and are tender enough to eat. Serve the bergamot sauce over the scapes.

Vegetable carpaccio make the perfect alternative to meat. They can be made with any vegetable you can eat raw – just thinly slice or peel into ribbons.

Courgette carpaccio with wood sorrel flowers

Simple and absolutely delicious. You can add an abundance of different flowers to this dish for additional flavour and colour too, such as borage and marigolds.

SERVES 4

6 courgettes

zest and juice of 1 lemon

1 tablespoon apple cider vinegar

1 small fresh red chilli, deseeded and thinly sliced

3 tablespoons oregano sprigs, leaves picked

drizzle of olive oil

a handful of mixed fresh wood sorrel flowers and leaves

salt and freshly ground black pepper

Rinse the courgettes, pat dry, then trim off the ends. Using a vegetable peeler, peel the courgettes (including the skins) into long, thin ribbons. Keep peeling until you get to the seeds in the middle, then discard these.

Place the courgette ribbons in a serving bowl, then add all the other ingredients, mixing the sorrel flowers and leaves through last, and seasoning with salt and pepper to taste. Cover and chill in the fridge for 30 minutes before serving.

Calendula, borage & fennel flower poached fish

If you are a vegan or prefer no dairy, simply switch out the milk for vegetable stock and the juice of a lemon. If like me you love it, you can switch the milk for cream.

SERVES 2

a good glug of olive oil
2 shallots, finely diced
700ml whole milk
small handful of fresh calendula flowers
small handful of fresh borage flowers
small handful of fresh fennel flowers
3 garlic cloves, smashed
½ teaspoon black peppercorns
2 skinless white fish fillets
salt and freshly ground black pepper

Heat the olive oil in a pan over a low heat. Add the shallots and cook for about 3–4 minutes until soft. Stir in the milk, half of the fennel flowers, the garlic and peppercorns. Bring the mixture to a medium simmer.

While the liquid heats up, season both sides of the fish fillets with salt and pepper. Reduce the heat to low and add the fish to the pan. Cover and cook for 8–10 minutes, or until the fish is opaque and flaky.

Remove the fish from the pan to serving bowls using a fish slice. Strain the poaching liquid, discarding the solids, then pour it over the fish. Garnish with the remaining flowers and serve with some fresh seasonal greens.

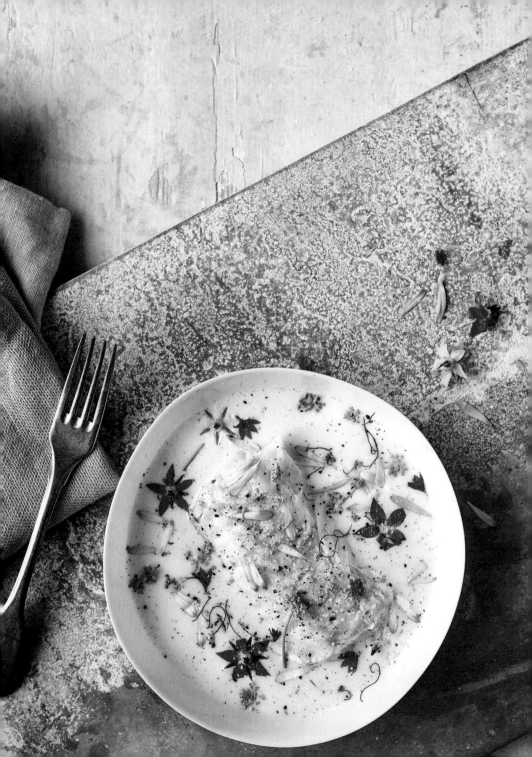

Dandelion soup

Dandelion is super dooper great for you. High in calcium and vitamin K, it cleanses your liver, fights infections and is high in antioxidants too. Eat soup. All of the soup.

SERVES 2

2 handfuls dandelion leaves, chopped
1 onion, diced
2 garlic cloves, finely chopped
2 celery sticks, chopped
knob of butter
480ml vegetable stock
1 handful dandelion petals, plus extra for garnishing
1 handful dandelion buds
zest of 1 lemon
rind from a piece of Parmesan cheese
240ml single cream, plus a little extra for drizzling
olive oil, for drizzling
salt and freshly ground black pepper

Blanch the dandelion leaves in a pan of boiling water for a few minutes, then plunge into iced water. Drain and set aside.

In a large pan, sauté the onion, garlic and celery in the butter until softened, about 5 minutes. Season with salt and pepper and then add the stock. Add all the remaining ingredients (including the blanched dandelion leaves), except the cream and olive oil, and bring to a simmer. Simmer, covered, for about 40 minutes, or until the vegetables are soft, stirring occasionally.

Remove the remains of the Parmesan rind and discard. Cool slightly, then pour the mixture into a blender and blend until smooth. Transfer back to the pan, stir in the cream, taste and season again. Reheat gently until hot (without boiling). Ladle into soup bowls and serve topped with more dandelion petals, a drizzle of olive oil and a little extra cream.

Resources

Below are just some of the fantastic edible flower suppliers you can source your ingredients and equipment from.

EDIBLE FLOWERS – UK & IRELAND
Nurtured in Norfolk
www.nurturedinnorfolk.co.uk
Maddocks Farm Organics
www.maddocksfarmorganics.co.uk
Greens of Devon
www.greensofdevon.com
Herbs Unlimited
www.herbsunlimited.co.uk
The Edible Flower Shop
www.theedibleflowershop.co.uk
The Flower Deli
www.theflowerdeli.co.uk

EDIBLE FLOWERS – AUSTRALIA
Petite Ingredient
www.petiteingredient.com.au
Sprout House Farms
www.sprouthousefarms.com.au
Pretty Produce
www.prettyproduce.com.au

BOTTLES, JARS, PACKAGING & DRIED INGREDIENTS
New Directions Australia
www.newdirections.com.au (delivery worldwide)
Amazon
www.amazon.co.uk

DRIED HERBS & FLOWERS – UK
Pestle Herbs
www.pestleherbs.co.uk

DRIED HERBS & FLOWERS – AUSTRALIA
Austral Herbs
www.australherbs.com.au

Index

Acknowledgements

Firstly to my family. My mum and dad have always supported me and I love that they sit in what my dad calls his 'proud chair' because of the path I am on. All I have ever wanted was to make them and my brothers proud. So to you my small family and the rest of my big extended family, especially its oh so wonderful leader my nan (and great grandmother Lil). To all of you, Sarah, Nigel, Paul, Mark, Kylie, Skye, Angie, Bec, Harry, Nicole, Yasmin, Sam, Teryn, Ashleigh, Caitlyn, Liam, Brad and Taylah and then the rest of our little family Emma, Koen and my godsons Charlie and Rory. You are all everything to me. As are you Damien, my love. Thank you for putting up with our home looking like a constant laboratory and test kitchen. To my friends who have supported me for decades. To Kyle. I have no words to express how grateful I am to you. To our new Octopus family, here is to a long journey making beautiful and meaningful books together. To my team. The A team. Tara, the most incredible Editor a girl could ask for. Your patience, generosity and passion for these next books made them what they are. Nassima. Thank you for making my recipes and creations come to life. I only hope we work on many a more things together. Rachel. No words can thank you enough for being the most incredible partner in crime styling these books and seeing inside my messy brain. You are so immensely talented and I am so grateful. Agathe, Laura and the rest of the team. High fives all round! To all of the people in my work world who have taught me so very much over the years. Thank you. There is no way I would be where I am without you teaching me everything I know. Last but not at all least, to all of you who bought this book. Massive gratitude from the bottom of my heart.